Kicking the Bear
Out of the Bedroom

Snoring & Sleep Apnea,
the Not-So-Silent Killers

Steve Wick

ISBN-13: 978-1539751885

ISBN-10: 1539751880

To my wife and daughter, who each in their own way,
propelled me on my journey.

DECEMBER 2016

STEVE —
Thanks for your continued support
and friendship throughout the years
through thick and thin! Here's to
a happy successful 2017 and a
Husky NATIONAL Championship!

[signature]

Table of Contents

INTRODUCTION

My name is Steve Wick and I'm a lucky guy. I have a beautiful, intelligent wife and nine-year-old daughter. We're happy and healthy and live busy, productive lives.

It wasn't always so.

I graduated with a degree in Economics from Seattle University in 1986. I had intended to go to law school, but too many extracurricular activities would have a negative impact on my GPA. It was suggested by my career guidance counselor, a month before graduation, that I might think about getting a job for a couple years before revisiting the law school idea.

I took her advice and began looking for a job. After several missteps, which may find their way into another book someday, I found a career.

Dentistry.

No, I'm not a dentist—but I've worked with literally thousands of them during the last twenty-five years. If my career counselor had told me I'd spend my career working with dentists, I would have told her she was crazy. The only dentist I knew at the time was my own, who cleaned my teeth every six months. You don't know what you don't know.

My first job was with a company that was relatively small at the time: Ivoclar Vivadent, headquartered in Liechtenstein. Ivoclar was, and still is, an innovative company. While I was there we were instrumental in changing the profession. We introduced tooth-colored composite fillings, which eventually replaced silver fillings in your teeth. We also introduced Empress Porcelain to the American market in the early 1990s, thereby creating the Esthetic Revolution in dentistry. Within five years every dentist in North America was a "cosmetic dentist."

I wouldn't trade those ten years for anything. I got to work chairside with some of the best dentists in the world as they used our products to change people's lives with beautiful smiles. Perhaps what I enjoyed most was teaching dentists something new. One of the greatest professional compliments I've ever received was when Ron, a dentist friend of mine, introduced me to one of his dental colleagues by saying, "Steve isn't a dentist, but he knows a lot more about dentistry than most dentists I know."

From changing people's lives, I moved on to quite literally saving people's lives, which turned out to be infinitely more rewarding. In 2004, I got the opportunity to help start a company, LED Medical Diagnostics. We took a technology, tissue fluorescence, developed by the British Columbia Cancer Agency, and commercialized it in the form of VELscope. VELscope allowed dentists to shine a special light in their patients' mouths and see abnormal tissue that they couldn't see with the naked eye. Tissue such as this has the potential to become malignant and transform to oral cancer.

I spent the next four years of my life crisscrossing the country lecturing dentists about the importance of early detection when dealing with abnormal tissue and oral cancer. It felt amazing to get emails and voicemails thanking me for introducing them to this technology. After each lecture I thought, "I think I might have saved a patient's life today."

What happened next is the reason I wrote this book.

I was unaware that throughout my career, and probably throughout my adolescence, I'd been suffering from an undiagnosed yet easily treated medical condition called "obstructive sleep apnea."

It came to my attention when my wife started complaining about my snoring. I began looking for a solution and was soon overwhelmed by what I uncovered. To make matters worse, in my case, like millions of other sufferers, the treatment offered turned out to be worse than the problem.

In this book you'll learn what I discovered:

1. Millions of people suffer from snoring and sleep apnea.
2. Most of these people are undiagnosed.
3. Untreated loud snoring can take ten years off of your life.
4. Untreated sleep apnea can lead to heart attack, stroke, high blood pressure, diabetes, and many other comorbidities.
5. Sleep apnea is easily diagnosed, treated, and managed once you know you have it.
6. CPAP isn't the only treatment option; there are several others.
7. Untreated sleep apnea costs the United States an estimated $150 billion a year in lost production, accidents, increased medical expenses, and additional societal costs.
8. Sleep apnea affects men, women, and children.
9. Sleep apnea in children is often misdiagnosed as ADHD, and not treating them for their sleep apnea can dramatically and negatively impact the rest of their lives.

With my new knowledge, I went from educator, to patient, and back to educator again.

As Paul Harvey used to famously say, "Now, here's the rest of the story..."

CHAPTER 1
The Rest of the Story

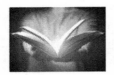 Today, 120 million Americans are suffering from a huge problem. It's practically an epidemic, and yet most of its sufferers don't even realize it—even you could have it. This problem can wreak havoc with your health, happiness, relationships and even financial well-being.

This is a "good news/bad news" story, however. The good news for many of us is that there's is a natural solution to this problem which is easy, free, and even enjoyable. The bad news is we actually have two problems.

The first problem is that we as a nation are chronically sleep-deprived. This includes men, women, and children. The second problem is that we don't know, or believe, this is even a problem.

This denial is strengthened by the culture we live in. We're taught from a young age that the more we work the further we'll get ahead. We're also taught to admire those hardworking, hard-charging individuals who can get by on only three or four hours of sleep a night. Those individuals who send us emails at two in the morning and proudly say with bravado, "I'll sleep when I'm dead!"

A normal night's sleep has a bad reputation in America, where sleep deprivation is worn like a Boy Scout merit badge. Our national motto, thanks to our industrious forefathers, might easily have been, "You snooze, you lose." Or, as Benjamin Franklin put it, "Up, sluggard, and waste not life; in the grave will be sleep enough." Thomas Edison, who guessed correctly that future Americans would sleep far less, declared, "Really, sleep is an absurdity, a bad habit."

This book wasn't written for those hard-charging, sleep-deprived, so-called "heroes." After all, it's their choice to do what they do, and nothing anyone can say will likely change their minds. No, this book was written for the millions of us who would like to get a good night's sleep but can't, for any number of reasons—most of which we're unaware.

There are over seventy sleep disorders currently recognized by the American Academy of Sleep Medicine. This book is going to focus on two of the more common sleep breathing disorders, snoring and obstructive sleep apnea.

I was one of the millions of ignorant sufferers of both these conditions—for decades! With the help of two individuals I admire greatly—Dr. Carrie Magnuson, a dentist whose practice solely treats patients with obstructive sleep apnea; and my friend Dr. Gandis Mazeika, a board-certified psychiatrist, neurologist, and sleep physician—I'll share with you my personal experience of identifying, coming to grips with, and getting treatment for, my sleep breathing disorders.

With the help of the doctors, whom I've enlisted to keep me honest and on track, we'll provide you, the reader, with a great amount of in-depth, up-to-date information regarding snoring and, more importantly, obstructive sleep apnea. These two conditions both contribute greatly to this nation's biggest under-appreciated and under-diagnosed epidemic: sleep deprivation.

Before we dive in too deep, however, let's start at the beginning.

CHAPTER 2
"How Much Sleep Do I Need? Why?"

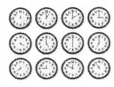 Sleep is a fundamental biological need just like food, water, and the air we breathe. In 1995, experiments conducted at the Sleep Research Laboratory at the University of Chicago showed that laboratory animals deprived of sleep actually die sooner than those deprived of food.

The first step on this journey is to answer your question: "How much sleep is enough?"

The National Sleep Foundation states that adults need 7–9 hours a night of restful sleep. Teenagers need at least 8–10 hours, adolescents need 9–11 hours, and newborn babies often require up to 17 hours of sleep a night.

Restful sleep restores the mind and body. It provides us with increased energy for the day ahead. There's nothing worse than having to tackle a busy day when you're exhausted due to a poor night's sleep. Sleep strengthens our immune system, which keeps us healthy. It allows us to safely discharge emotions through dreaming. It improves our cognitive learning skills. It improves our memories through consolidation. Think about all the thousands of things you're exposed to throughout the day, everything from a gum wrapper on the ground to that new project your boss just gave you. During sleep the memories and thoughts that aren't important are discarded, while the important stuff is cataloged and put into the right filing cabinet in our brain.

A good night's sleep also helps us cope with the everyday stresses of life. When we're sleep-deprived, we wake up cranky and often spend the day in a fog. Easy tasks become challenging. Our minds wander, preventing us from focusing on the job at hand. Our coping skills are diminished, which may cause us to overreact, resulting in negative consequences.

For me personally, 1:00 p.m. couldn't come fast enough every day. I'm lucky, in that I'm either working out of my home office or traveling for business. While working at home, my couch would call my name every afternoon at one o'clock, for my half-hour nap. When I was on the road, I'd schedule my meetings around my "downtime" whenever possible. I doubt if this ritual would have gone over very well working in a traditional office environment, but it worked for me, for a time.

Although I was constantly tired, I told myself this was normal. I worked hard and played hard. "Everyone's tired, get over it," I'd tell myself. On long driving trips I'd experience "white line fever," as truckers call it—that experience where your mind wanders while you're driving, but somehow you get where you were going without even realizing it. If I'd start to nod off, I'd turn the radio up and roll down the windows. "The colder the better, just stay awake," I would say to myself, "we're almost there." I'd promise myself that I'd sleep in on the weekend to "catch up" on my sleep.

Little did I know how dangerous these little tricks truly were.

CHAPTER 3
How Much Sleep Are We Getting?

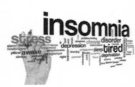 A recent National Sleep Foundation poll found that adults now average 6.9 hours of sleep each night, slightly less than the low end of the recommended amount. Additionally, a Sleep in America poll reported that more people now say they are sleeping less than six hours on weekdays (16% in 2016 vs. 13% in 1998) as well as on weekends (10% in 2016 vs. 8% in 1998).

Remember those workaholics who try and get by on three or four hours a night? Consider the following: getting just two to three hours of sleep a few nights in a row can have the same effect as pulling an all-nighter—yet it's something that many Americans routinely do. A National Institute of Justice study, published in March 2009, showed that 24 hours without sleep is equivalent to a blood alcohol level of .10, which is above the legal limit for operating a motor vehicle in all fifty states.

Just like a credit card or a mortgage, sleep debt eventually has to be repaid. And the more you add to it, the bigger your negative balance.

Sleeping in on the weekends (a common practice) is one way that you might try to combat a shortage of weeknight sleep, but it's not a very good strategy. If you're under-sleeping by even an hour every night during the week, you'll end up with a sleep debt of five hours by the time Saturday rolls around. By trying to deposit those five hours over the weekend by sleeping in, you'll throw off your regular sleep schedule for the following week.

Here's one last wake-up call regarding sleep deprivation:

Sleep deprivation has been used as a form of interrogation and torture for centuries. Sleep deprivation reduces our psychological resistance and reduces the body's ability to resist pain. The National Academy of Science published research conducted in 1996 on false confessions during criminal interrogations, which it turns out may be more common than we realize. False confessions account for approximately 15–20% of all wrongful convictions in the United States. Sleep deprivation may lead a person to accept responsibility and confess to something that never happened. Participants in the study were instructed to complete multiple computer tasks and were repeatedly warned not to press the "Escape" key, as it would cause the loss of data. Participants were then divided into two groups who either slept all night in a sleep lab or were kept awake. The following morning, all participants were asked to sign a summary statement of what had occurred in the lab, and were falsely accused of pressing "Escape." After just one request, those that were sleep-deprived were 4.5 times more likely to sign that they were guilty of pressing the "Escape" key than those who'd had a full night's sleep.

As time went, on I continually adapted to my own sleep deprivation and the consequences, until one day I'd had enough and couldn't take it anymore. As I began to take a more proactive approach to my lack of sleep, I found out that lack of sleep wasn't my problem, but was in fact a symptom of a much bigger problem that I didn't know I had. A problem that, left untreated, could lead to any number of serious health issues including heart attack and death.

CHAPTER 4
Getting a Good Night's Sleep

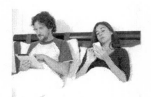 Before we discuss the scary stuff, I want to introduce you to a concept called "proper sleep hygiene."

The term "sleep hygiene" refers to a series of habits and rituals that can improve your ability to fall asleep and stay asleep. Board-certified sleep physicians recommend following a series of common-sense healthy sleep habits to promote better sleep. They consist of the following, published by the American Sleep Association:

1. Go to bed at the same time and wake up at the same time every day. Ideally, your schedule will remain the same every night of the week (plus or minus twenty minutes).
2. Avoid naps if possible. When we take naps, it decreases the amount of sleep that we need the next night. This can cause sleep disruptions or fragmentation and difficulty initiating sleep. This cycle may then lead to insomnia.
3. Don't stay in bed, awake, for more than five to ten minutes. This time is called "sleep onset." If you find your mind racing or worrying about not being able to go to sleep in the middle of the night, get out of bed and sit in a chair in the dark. Let your mind race while sitting in the chair. Wait until your mind settles down and you're sleepy, then go back to bed. If this happens several times during the night, that's OK. Just maintain your regular wake time, and try and avoid naps.
4. The bed was designed for two things: sleep and intimacy. Nothing else. The average adult spends a third of their life in bed. Invest in the best mattress and bed linens you can afford. Most mattress stores have a minimum of a thirty-day return policy. Take advantage of it if you need to in order to find your perfect mattress.

5. In a perfect world, we wouldn't have televisions in the bedroom, but many of us do. Turn the TV off when you're ready for bed. The blue light emitted by televisions creates another problem. Blue light inhibits the release of melatonin and interrupts your natural circadian rhythm. Melatonin is a hormone made by the pineal gland, a small gland in the brain. It helps control your sleep and wake cycles. It dips and rises at different times of the day, and tells you when it's time to go to sleep and when it's time to wake up. Your circadian rhythm is your internal biological clock, which also regulates sleep and awake time. Your internal clock can be negatively influenced by the amount of light that is present in your bedroom.

6. The same thing holds true for laptops and tablets. They both emit blue light, decreasing melatonin and altering your circadian rhythm. Whatever you're shopping for on eBay will still be there in the morning!

7. Put your cell phone away too, as it emits blue light as well. But that's the least of its problems. If your job requires you to be "on call," put your phone on vibrate if you must. Wouldn't you rather deal with all of those "important" emails in the morning when you're rested?

8. If there's a book that you just can't put down, get up. Leave the bedroom and find a comfortable chair to sit in. After thirty minutes of reading you'll be ready to put the book down and go to bed. This also works if you're lying in bed trying to fall asleep. Get up, go to your favorite chair, and read for a bit. (As an added bonus, there are special light bulbs available that don't emit blue light. Use one of these in the lamp by your reading chair for best results.)

9. Your bedroom should be quiet and cool. If you live in an area where external outside noise is a problem, background "white noise" like a fan might prove relaxing. Set your bedroom thermostat at a comfortable temperature. A little cooler is better. It makes that bed look and feel cozy and inviting. Your bedroom should also be dark. Close the curtains and turn off bright lights.

10. If you have pets, consider keeping them out of the bedroom. This may be difficult, but a rested pet owner is a happy pet owner.

11. Remember when your mother used to say, "Don't go to bed on a full stomach"? She was right! Don't eat heavy meals after 6:00 p.m. Heavy meals need time to be digested properly.

12. Don't consume caffeinated beverages after noon. The effects of caffeine can last for hours after consumption. Caffeine can fragment sleep and make falling asleep difficult. Remember that soda, tea, and even some foods contain caffeine as well.

13. Cigarettes, alcohol, and over-the-counter medications may cause fragmented sleep as well. Nicotine in cigarettes is a stimulant, which prohibits sleep. Alcohol may help you fall asleep, but it interrupts or fragments your sleep later in the night. Check with your pharmacist regarding any side effects that may affect your sleep in any way. Include all prescription or over-the-counter medications you may be taking.

14. Exercise before 2:00 p.m. every day. Exercise promotes continuous sleep, but avoid exercise before bedtime. Rigorous exercise circulates endorphins throughout your body. Endorphins make you feel energized, which is great during the day, but not as good right before bed.

15. Have a comfortable pre-bedtime routine. Take a warm bath or shower. Brush your teeth and wash your face. Meditate to quiet your mind before you lay down. Whatever you do, make it the same routine. Your mind will begin to associate it with sleep.

I've added one more addition to the list that works for me:

16. As children, we were told that if all else fails, try "counting sheep." Why sheep? It didn't work for me. I "play golf" in my head instead. When I was growing up I played golf every day all summer at our local course, literally hundreds

of rounds. When I can't sleep, I imagine myself standing on the, first tee of my home course. I then proceed to play a round of golf in my mind, imagining myself hitting each shot exactly where it needs to go. First hole, par five, hit a drive up the right side of the fairway. Second shot, three wood toward the left side of the fairway, giving me a better approach angle to the green. You get the idea. I very seldom make it past the seventh hole, but I'm always at even par.

Another calming trick is to make a mental list of the things you love, in alphabetical order. Disclaimer: some letters are harder than others. If you can't think of something, skip it and come back later if you haven't already fallen asleep. My guess is you won't make it through the alphabet. Sweet dreams!

CHAPTER 5
I Still Had a Problem or Three

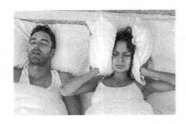 My real problems started about five years into my happy marriage. I suddenly started showing signs of "bruised rib syndrome." This is a non-medical condition caused by a bed partner who doesn't appreciate your snoring.

How many of you reading this book have been accused or have known someone else guilty of snoring? I'd bet that every one of you can name someone. I grew up in a family with a brother and sister and six close cousins. Thanksgiving was always at Grandpa and Grandma's house. When we were young we all made a pact: whoever woke up first had to promise to wake up everyone else so we could all listen to Grandpa snoring. What fun we had—you could hear him from every room in the house, upstairs or down. We'd laugh and then take turns trying to out-snore him between fits of laughter.

This story is not about my childhood, however, so back to my bruised rib syndrome. I'm not sure what I was doing during our first five years of marriage, but according to my wife, I now snored quite loudly and annoyingly. The funny thing was that when she'd wake me up with a shove and a snarl, I'd say "I can't be snoring ... I wasn't even asleep!"

That's the fundamental problem with snoring: the snorer doesn't know and may not care that they're snoring. They should, for a number of good reasons.

Here are some startling statistics from the National Sleep Foundation (NSF). The NSF estimates that 90 million Americans have a snoring problem, and that 45% of all adults snore at least occasionally. Snoring can in some cases, over time, lead to permanent hearing loss for you and/or your bed partner. A loud snorer is often over the limit of 90 decibels, a level at which the Occupational Safety and Health Administration (OSHA) requires hearing protection. 90 dB is the noise level of a blender turned on high! Of greater concern, however, is that it's also estimated that 80% of couples with a snoring partner sleep in separate rooms. This statistic gives credence to a recent article in the *Ladies' Home Journal* that called a snoring spouse the third most common problem leading to divorce.

What causes snoring, you might be wondering? Good question. The easiest way to describe what's causing all the racket is to use a garden hose analogy.

Imagine yourself out watering your garden on a beautiful summer evening. You've stretched the hose as far as it will go but you can't quite reach the last flower bed. What do you do? You put your thumb over the end of the hose, partially blocking the water. What happens? The same amount of water traveling through a smaller opening moves faster, thereby going farther. Now think of your airway as the garden hose. While we're awake and upright the muscles in our neck, throat, and mouth remain tight, which keeps our airway (hose) wide open. But when we lay down and begin to fall asleep, something happens. Our muscles relax, and gravity takes over. Slowly our lower jaw begins to slide back and our airway begins to narrow. When the same amount of air moves through a narrower opening, just like the water in the hose, it speeds up. Air, moving faster, causes turbulence. Turbulence causes the soft tissue in our mouths and throats to vibrate. Vibrating tissue is noisy.

There you have it—snoring!

Snoring can be problematic for friends, family, and in extreme cases the neighbors, but what about the person making all the noise, the snorer?

An article published in the *American Academy of Sleep Medicine Journal* in March, 2008, states: "Compared to non-snorers, loud snorers have 67% greater likelihood of having a stroke, a 40% greater likelihood of having high blood pressure, and a 34% greater likelihood of having a heart attack." Additionally, the *New England Journal of Medicine* (2005: 352: 1138–1145) shared research showing that the life expectancy of an untreated snorer was up to ten years shorter than a non-snorer. Lastly, and most important of all, loud snoring is a primary indicator of someone suffering from obstructive sleep apnea.

CHAPTER 6
OSA: "What Is It and Who Has It?"

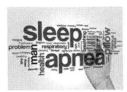 To explain obstructive sleep apnea, or OSA, we'll use the garden hose example again.

Imagine, if you will, that no one wakes you up while you're snoring. Your muscles continue to relax and your lower jaw continues to fall back until your airway totally collapses, causing airflow to stop completely.

We all know that we need to breathe to live, so you might be wondering what happens next.

When the brain realizes that we aren't getting oxygen anymore, alarm bells begin to sound and our brain sends a message to the body, saying, "Wake up, dummy, we're not breathing and we're gonna die!" A shot of adrenaline is sent to the heart and our system is flooded with a hormone called cortisol.

Adrenaline is a hormone secreted by the adrenal glands, especially during times of stress. It increases the rate of blood circulation, breathing, and prepares the muscles for exertion. Cortisol is known as the "fight-or-flight hormone" and can come in handy in certain unpleasant stressful situations. Think about how your body feels when you're scared—that rush is a combination of adrenaline and cortisol.

When we should be restfully sleeping, our mind and body feel like we're running on a treadmill, due to these infusions of adrenalin and cortisol.

OSA can vary greatly in severity. Sleep apnea is measured using an AHI, or Apnea Hypopnea Index. This index measures the number of times each and every hour throughout the night that an individual stops breathing for a minimum of ten seconds.

An AHI of less than five is considered normal.

An AHI between five and fifteen is considered mild sleep apnea.

Moderate sleep apnea is a score of fifteen to thirty times an hour.

Lastly, we have severe obstructive sleep apnea. This is where an individual stops breathing for a minimum of ten seconds thirty or more times an hour, every hour, all night long. With each episode comes a shot of adrenaline and cortisol.

Sound like fun?

The number of OSA sufferers in the United States is open for debate due to the lack of recent independent studies, but I'll share with you some things that we do know. In a 1993 study published in the *New England Journal of Medicine*, it was estimated that 24% of adult males and 9% of adult females suffered from OSA. Sorry, guys, but gender as well as age and obesity are contributing factors to developing OSA. The percentages quoted in this study correlates to approximately 18 million Americans suffering from OSA, with the worldwide number of sufferers surpassing 100 million individuals. The problem with these numbers is that the data was published in 1993. Between 1993 and 2016 what do we know, as fact, happened in the United States?

1) We've all gotten older—it's just a fact of life.

2) Most of us have gotten bigger—look in the mirror.

The Endowment for Human Development (www.edh.org) measures obesity trends in the United States. They reported that in 1993—the same year the OSA prevalence study was published—approximately 15% of adults throughout the United States were classified as "obese," which is a body mass index (BMI) greater than thirty, or approximately thirty pounds overweight, for a 5'4" person. By 2006, the last year that data was available, that number had risen from 15% to 27%, an average increase of   approximately one percent a year. Given this one-percent annual increase, it's reasonable to assume that obesity in America has increased to 37% over the last ten years.

What do these statistics suggest about the number of OSA suffers currently?

A new study which was based in Switzerland and published last year in the *Lancet Respiratory Medicine Journal* found that the number of women suffering from OSA had climbed from 9% in 1993 to 23.4% in 2013. The number of men affected by OSA had also increased, rising from 24% in 1993 to 49.7% in 2013.

It seems reasonable that the same increases found in Switzerland would also be found in the United States and elsewhere. If this is the case, the number of OSA suffers in the United States has increased from 18 million in 1993 to 36.5 million in 2013.

One more disturbing fact before we move own: It is commonly accepted in the medical community that 90% of OSA sufferers are undiagnosed and unaware that they have a serious medical problem.

Why is this?

Physicians don't ask.

The article "Evolution of Sleep Disorders in the Primary Care Setting," published in Vol. 7, No. 1, 2011, of the *Journal of Clinical Sleep Medicine*, asked primary care physicians:

"How often do you ask your patients about how well they sleep?"

Physicians self-reported that they asked 29% of their patients. When asked why they didn't ask a higher percentage of patients, they gave these three main reasons:

- Lack of awareness
- Limited time during appointment

- Lack of reimbursement (insurance coverage)
- High demand in addressing patients' immediate concerns

Another unfortunate fact about obstructive sleep apnea is that there is no cure. It's a medical condition that can be managed for a lifetime, but very seldom does it ever go away.

CHAPTER 7
My Story and More

 In Chapter 2, I admitted to afternoon naps on the couch.

Needing an afternoon nap isn't normal for people who get a good nights' sleep. I was suffering from excessive day-time sleepiness (EDS), another symptom of OSA. My snoring Grandpa from Chapter 5 also suffered from EDS. Remember him?

Christmas time was also a time for our extended family to get together. One year, the whole family celebrated Christmas in Spokane at my aunt and uncle's house. With nine kids and eight adults under one roof, it was a mad house. Christmas morning came and went and Grandpa decided it was time to head home before it got dark. He got into his Cadillac and pulled out of the drive way, prepared for a three-hour drive home.

Driving through the wheat fields of Eastern Washington can be numbingly boring. It's definitely "cruise-control country." Halfway through the trip, Grandpa, with the cruise control set on sixty, fell asleep.

Luckily, the car drifted off the road on a section with a flat shoulder. His car continued twenty-five yards into the muddy wheat field until the tires began to lose traction.

Sometime later a State Patrolman, not believing what he was seeing, stopped his car and walked out into the field and up to the driver's side window. He looked inside and saw my grandfather, snoring away while his back wheels continued to spin in the mud.

Years later, I'd still find myself dozing at the wheel during long trips. On one occasion, I started in the left-hand lane only to wake up seconds later having drifted over two lanes to the right. On another occasion, knowing that I was tired, I got off the freeway intending to find a place to park and take a quick power-nap. Imagine my embarrassment when I was awakened by a knock on my window. I'd fallen asleep at the stop sign at the end of the off-ramp. The driver behind me had gotten out of his car and walked up to check on me.

EDS can often be identified by taking a simple quiz called the Epworth Sleepiness Scale, or ESS. The Epworth Sleepiness Scale was introduced in 1991 by Dr. Murray Johns, of Epworth Hospital in Melbourne, Australia. I've included the ESS quiz at the end of this chapter.

Believe it or not, EDS wasn't my wake-up call—Restless Leg Syndrome (RLS) was. I'd never heard of RLS, but I knew that whenever I was tired and sat or laid down, I had an uncontrollable urge to move my legs. When I was young, my mom would joke that I had "high-performance legs" whenever they'd begin to twitch. As an adult, it was no longer funny. Sometimes the only way that I could fall asleep once my legs began moving was to get up in the middle of the night and walk around the house for an hour. As I got older it got progressively worse. So much so that I could time the twitching. Every twelve or thirteen seconds I'd have to move my legs. This would go on for hours.

Salvation came in 2005.

I was watching television one evening when a commercial for the new drug Requip came on. It was the first time I'd ever heard of restless leg syndrome, but based on the commercial I was sure I had it. I made an appointment to see our family doctor as soon as possible. The following week, when she walked into the examination room I immediately said, "I have restless leg syndrome and I want to try Requip."

Luckily for me, she had a basic understanding of sleep disorders. Many primary care physicians don't.

She replied, "Steve, number one: you don't get to self-diagnose in my office; and number two: you don't get to self-prescribe medication." She explained to me that RLS was often associated with OSA, and that I would have to see a sleep specialist and rule out OSA before she'd prescribe Requip.

She proceeded to describe OSA to me as I've described it to you in Chapter 6.

I was sure I wasn't suffering from OSA and told her so, adding defensively, "I'm a light sleeper."

She persisted that I see the sleep specialist. I wanted those pills, so I made an appointment.

Epworth Sleepiness Scale (ESS)

How likely are you to doze off during one of the following situations?

0 = WOULD NEVER DOZE OFF

1 = SLIGHT CHANCE OF DOZING

2 = MODERATE CHANCE OF DOZING

3 = HIGH CHANCE OF DOZING

1. Sitting and reading?
2. Watching television?
3. Sitting inactive in a public place (meeting, theatre, etc.)?
4. As a passenger in a car for an hour without a break?
5. Lying down to rest in the afternoon whenever circumstances permit?
6. Sitting and talking to someone?
7. Sitting quietly after a meal without alcohol?
8. In a car, while stopped in traffic for a few minutes?

TOTAL SCORE:

A score of 11 or greater puts you at high risk for OSA.

CHAPTER 8
The Sleep Test

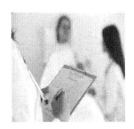

Three weeks later (you wouldn't believe how busy sleep doctors are), I was able to get in to see the sleep specialist.

I repeated to him what I'd told my primary care doctor: "I have restless leg syndrome and I want Requip." For good measure I added, "I'm also a light sleeper and I don't have sleep apnea."

He simply replied, "Why don't we find out for sure?"

He had me take another questionnaire called the STOPBang to help determine if I might be suffering from OSA. I've included the STOPBang questionnaire at the end of this chapter.

The doctor looked at my STOPBang answers, as well as my ESS score, and concluded that I was indeed at high risk for obstructive sleep apnea. He explained to me that the only sure way to determine if I was a sufferer was to take part in a sleep study.

I agreed half-heartedly, after further homework. First I wanted to find out all I could about sleep studies. Second, I wanted to know the signs and symptoms associated with sleep apnea and what factors might make it better or worse. To my computer and Google I went.

This is what I discovered:

Topic number one: sleep studies. Sleep studies come in two flavors. The traditional sleep study is called "polysomnography," or PSG for short. This test is administered in a hospital or private sleep lab. Prior to going to sleep, a number of electrodes are attached at different points on your body. These electrodes record your brain waves, the oxygen level in your blood, your heart rate, limb movements, respiratory effort (how hard you try to breathe), snoring, and eye movement. In addition to the electrodes, you are watched while you sleep via closed circuit television, which is monitored by a Registered Polysomnographic Technologist (RPSGT) throughout your sleep study.

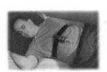 The second option, which has become much more prevalent in recent years due to its significantly lower cost, is the home sleep test—HST for short. The HST is a small machine that the patient takes home for the night. It's attached to the body in much the same way as a PSG and measures some of the same things. HSTs are limited somewhat by the fact that they don't monitor as many vital signs as a PSG does, and a RPSGT is not present in your bedroom to monitor your sleep.

If you find yourself in need of a sleep study, the sleep doctor will determine which type you get based on your health history. Due to my RLS concerns, the sleep doctor required that my sleep study be monitored, so I was scheduled for a PSG the next Friday night. He let me know that he'd score my test and send the results back to my doctor for her to review with me.

I didn't care what I had to do at this point. Anything to get my pills. I felt like an addict, even though I'd never even tried the drug!

When I got home that night I immediately Googled "PSG," which only brought me to a French soccer club with the same initials.

I then tried "Polysomnography" and immediately regretted it. Right there on YouTube was my worst nightmare, depicted in living color. As I watched, fascinated, I kept repeating to myself, "I need the pills, I need the pills, I need the pills ..."

The second topic—signs and symptoms of OSA—was well addressed with the two questionnaires I'd been given, but I found some additional information. As far as my signs and symptoms were concerned:

1. *Snoring?* Yep, according to my wife.
2. *Tired during the day?* That went without saying.
3. *Observed having stopped breathing during sleep?* Once this process began, my wife became much more observant, and stated that yes, she had witnessed me stop breathing while asleep.
4. *High blood pressure?* Thankfully not.
5. *BMI greater than 35?* Nope, but I could stand to lose some weight. If you Google "BMI calculator," you can calculate your own body mass index.
6. *50 years of age or older?* Just barely.
7. *Neck size greater than 17 inches?* Just barely.
8. *Male?* Yes.
9. *Suffering from morning headaches?* Yes.
10. *Waking up with a dry mouth or sore throat?* Sometimes.
11. *Experiencing mood changes, such as depression or irritability?* Sure, on occasion.
12. *Excessive nocturnal urination (getting up and having to go to the bathroom more than once a night)?* What did 3–4 times a night mean, I wondered?
13. *Decreased libido?* Compared to what? I wasn't in my twenties any more.
14. *Nocturnal bruxism (grinding and clenching of teeth during the night)?* Again, according to my wife, guilty as charged.

Lastly, although it didn't apply to me, I found out that certain medications can make sleep apnea worse.

They fall into three categories:

Benzodiazepines are medications prescribed to relieve anxiety. Some of them work as muscle relaxants or are used to treat seizures. They can also cause sleepiness. Some of the brand names include Xanax, Klonopin, and Valium.

Opiates (sometimes called "opioids" or "narcotics"), are a class of medications used to treat pain. They often cause sleepiness that can cause increased respiratory pauses, irregular breathing, and shallow breaths. Examples of opiates include Hydrocodone, Oxycodone, Codeine, Morphine, and Fentanyl. Fentanyl contributed to the recent deaths of both Michael Jackson and Prince.

Lastly are barbiturates. Barbiturates are used for sedation, but because of serious side effects, including the risk of dependence and withdrawal, they have largely been phased out as sleep aids. The most common example is Phenobarbital.

Based on my research, the odds were pretty high that I had obstructive sleep apnea.

Too soon for my liking, Friday evening arrived. Fortified by a couple cocktails, I showed up for my sleep study. (I later found out this was a *bad idea*! Remember alcohol consumption and sleep fragmentation, in Chapter 4.)

The technician explained the process to me, I got in my pajamas, the wires were hooked up, and I laid down and tried to go to sleep.

Needless to say, this was not a particularly peaceful night. Between wrapping myself up in all the wires I was attached to, constantly detaching myself to get up and go to the bathroom and then reattaching myself, I was sure the night was a waste. I was awake and ready to get out of that place at 6:00 a.m. the next morning. Luckily for me, the sleep technician said he'd gotten enough information, during the five minutes or so that I imagined I'd been asleep, to allow the doctor to provide a diagnosis. He also informed me that the doctor would probably want me back soon for something he called a follow-up CPAP titration study. I didn't wait around to find out what that might be.

The following is the STOPBang questionnaire mentioned earlier. The STOPBang was developed in 2008 by Dr. Frances Chung at the University of Toronto as a pre-surgery screening tool. As you might imagine, it is extremely important for the anesthesiologist to know if the patient they are about to put to sleep suffers from OSA. The STOPBang questions tackle the various areas that predispose a person to sleep apnea. If a patient positively responds to three or more questions, they are considered to be at a moderate risk level for OSA; a score of five or more positive responses puts a patient at high risk for OSA. Various studies since 2008 have validated the STOPBang questionnaire's accuracy for predicting OSA. It, along with the Epworth Sleepiness Scale, remains the most used screening tool to this day.

STOPBang Questionnaire

S: Do you Snore loudly (louder than talking or loud enough to be heard through closed doors)?

T: Do you often feel Tired, fatigued, or sleepy during the day?

O: Has anyone Observed you not breathing during sleep?

P: Do you have or have you been treated for high blood Pressure?

B: Is your Body mass index (BMI) greater than 35kg/m² (Google "BMI calculator")?

A: Is your Age more than 50 years old?

N: Is your Neck circumference greater than 17 inches men, 16 inches women?

G: Is your Gender male?

If you answered "**YES**" to 3–5 of these questions, you are at **MODERATE RISK** for OSA. 5 or more "**YES**" answers put you in the **HIGH RISK** category.

CHAPTER 9
Diagnosis & Treatment

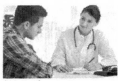 Three days later I got a call from my doctor that my test results were back. I made an appointment for the next day and thought about my pills until my legs finally stopped jumping at 3:00 a.m. and I could fall asleep.

The next day my doctor walked into the examination room with a big smile on her face.

I asked, "Good news?"

She smiled again and said, "I was just remembering when we first started this conversation and you told me you were a light sleeper. Turns out you were right!"

"I remember," I replied, a bit dryly. "What about my pills?"

"We'll get to that, but first we need to review your sleep study," she continued. "It turns out that in addition to your self-diagnosed restless leg syndrome, you're also suffering from severe obstructive sleep apnea."

Remember the definition of severe OSA in Chapter 6? Severe sleep apnea is a patient with an AHI of thirty or higher.

My doctor said, "You're not a light sleeper—you're not sleeping at all! Your AHI is a 73, which means that you stop breathing 73 times an hour for a minimum of ten seconds at a time, every hour, all night long. Not only will I write you a prescription for the pills for your RLS, but I'm also sending you to get a CPAP."

I left her office, stopped by the pharmacy, got my pills, and went home.

My wife asked me over dinner that night about my test results. I said, "I got my pills and I also need something called a CPAP, whatever that is."

I took my pill later that evening, and for the first time that I could remember my legs behaved and I slept through the night—if you don't count the three or four rib-shots I got from my wife.

Something still wasn't right.

CHAPTER 10
What's with the Mask?

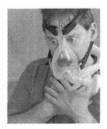 The next morning, I Googled "CPAP," and Tom Cruise from the movie *Top Gun* glared back at me with his fighter pilot mask on. (Lesson learned: don't Google acronyms!)

As I continued to read, the excitement of finally getting my pills began to wear off. What I found out was this:

CPAP, which stands for Continuous Positive Air Pressure, can best be described as a vacuum cleaner running in reverse. The air is blowing out rather than sucking in. Now put the end of the vacuum cleaner hose in your mouth and wrap your lips around it. The air blowing down your throat keeps your airway from collapsing while you sleep.

Sounds appealing, doesn't it?

Even with this new information I was willing to give CPAP a try, because it was the only way my doctor would keep refilling my prescription for my RLS medicine, which was allowing me after years of discomfort to finally sleep at night. Don't get me wrong— CPAP is considered the *gold standard* for treating OSA. In fact, it is 100% effective.

The problem is in the fine print.

Compliance, or usage, is the hidden problem with CPAP therapy. There are any number of reasons for CPAP noncompliance, among them skin irritation around the mask, rhinitis (nasal inflammation that results in a runny nose), congestion, nasal itch, sneezing, drying out of the mouth—not to mention the noise and inconvenience associated with sleeping attached to a machine via a hose and mask. Various studies have shown CPAP compliance at or below 50% after two years.

What does this really mean in numbers?

ResMed and Respironics are the two largest CPAP manufacturers in the world. Combined, they sell 125,000 CPAPs a month in the United States alone. If 50% of CPAP-treated patients discontinue use after only two years, that means that every month over 60,000 people who know they're sick and were willing to try sleeping with a mask on their faces have given up on treatment.

CPAP, for them, is worse than sleep apnea.

That means that 720,000 patients a year discontinue treatment of this life-threatening medical condition. And they don't believe—or, worse yet, weren't even told—that there are any other treatment options.

The truth is, like most medical conditions, there *are* other options. We'll discuss those later in the book, but let me tell you about my CPAP experience first.

CHAPTER 11
Me and My CPAP

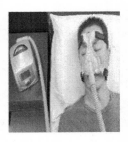 On the insistence of my doctor, I went back to the sleep doctor for my CPAP.

As it turns out, I was getting a little ahead of myself again. Remember the morning after my first sleep study when the technician mentioned a follow-up CPAP titration study? Well, it came up again when I tried to make an appointment to pick up my new toy.

It turns out that before I could get the CPAP that I didn't want, I'd have to partake in another PSG sleep study, and this one contained a new twist. I would repeat the same process I'd gone through three weeks earlier, but this time I'd be using a CPAP machine. The technician would monitor my sleep throughout the night and periodically adjust the air pressure on my CPAP to optimize my airflow. The idea was to find the ideal air pressure to treat my sleep apnea without blowing me out of bed.

Sounded to me like more fun than a barrel of monkeys. I scheduled myself for another Friday-night sleep study at the end of the week.

If you thought the first study had been miserable, let me tell you— the second beat it hands down. Everything—the wires, the camera, the technician—remained the same, but this time they added the mask.

The first time you try and sleep with a mask on your face is an interesting experience, to say the least. Luckily, I made the best of an uncomfortable situation and fell asleep just long enough for my CPAP to be titrated.

The next day, I got dressed and was sent down the hall to the Durable Medical Equipment (DME) coordinator, who fitted me with my own fancy machine, gave me a few instructions which I promptly forgot, and sent me home with my very own CPAP.

The first couple of nights I'd tear my mask off in the middle of the night and find it laying on the floor in the morning. As the weeks progressed, it stayed on a bit longer each night. Once I got used to the mask, however, I kept getting tangled up in the hose.

I realized after about ninety days that those noncompliant patients might be right. Untreated sleep apnea was better than sleeping with a CPAP mask strapped to my face. I silently joined their ranks and put my CPAP in the closet, hoping that the CPAP fairies would take it away.

Like most people with OSA whom I've spoken to over the last six years, my sleep doctor didn't tell me there were any other options other than CPAP, and like many people, the last thing I wanted to do was to go back to my doctor and say that I'd failed treatment. I had my pills, and was therefore sleeping better.

What was a little snoring and a few bruised ribs, anyway?

CHAPTER 12
The Wake-Up Call & Reality Check

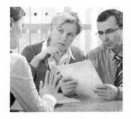 My wake-up call came six months later.

Arriving home from a week-long business trip, I walked into our newly remodeled home to the smell of my gourmet wife breaking in our new kitchen.

She said, "Let me pour you a cocktail and you can take a shower while I finish dinner."

I thought to myself, "What did I do to deserve this?" I kissed her, thanked her, grabbed my drink, and headed to the shower.

After dinner was over and we were settling in for the evening, she said, "I have one more thing for you," and handed me an envelope.

I opened it, not knowing what to expect, and read:

Dear Daddy,

My name is Sidney.

I looked at my wife, confused, and asked, "Who's Daddy and who's Sidney?"

But as the words came out of my mouth I realized that she was telling me that she was pregnant and we were about to become parents with our first child.

Becoming a parent, or at least knowing that it's inevitable, changes things. You realize that you're going to be responsible for another human being beside yourself.

The responsible thing to do was to get life insurance, which neither of us had ever had or needed before. We filled out the paperwork, sent it in, and forgot about it until our insurance broker called. He stated matter-of-factly that they wouldn't insure me.

I couldn't understand it. I was only 46. I didn't smoke. I didn't have high blood pressure. I didn't drink excessively. I could stand to lose twenty pounds, but I worked out semi-regularly. What was the problem?

My insurance agent asked me, "Have you ever been diagnosed with obstructive sleep apnea?"

I answered, "Yes."

His next question was the deal breaker.

"Are you currently using the CPAP that was prescribed to you a year ago?"

I sheepishly replied that no, I had given up on my CPAP treatment.

That's when he hit me right between the eyes.

"The reason we can't insure you is that you are going to die. You have sleep apnea and you're not treating it."

CHAPTER 13
I Feel Fine. How Bad Can It Be, Anyway?

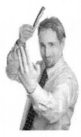 I figured that the only reason an insurance company wouldn't take my money was that they knew something that I didn't, and I was going to find out what it was.

It turns out it was a lot of things, and they were called "comorbidities."

Comorbidity is the presence of one or more additional diseases or disorders occurring simultaneously with a primary disease, which in my case was OSA. The comorbidities associated with OSA can be divided into four categories: Cardiovascular, Cerebrovascular, Metabolic Issues, and Societal Costs.

Cardiovascular disease generally refers to conditions affecting the blood vessels and/or heart. Cardiovascular issues directly related to OSA include high blood pressure, heart attack, cardiac arrhythmia (irregular heartbeat), erectile dysfunction, and frequent nocturnal urination.

Additional research has confirmed the increased risk of having a heart attack when additional health factors are considered. The study, published in the *Lancet Medical Journal* in 1990, showed that obesity increases your risk of having a heart attack by a factor of seven. You are eight times more likely to have a heart attack if you have high blood pressure, and eleven times more likely if you smoke.

What would you guess the number is for OSA?

If you suffer from untreated OSA, you are twenty-three times more likely to have a heart attack than someone without sleep apnea.

The risk is almost the same as someone who is obese, has high blood pressure, and smokes all at the same time!

One last mention of my grandfather: knowing what I know now, there's no doubt in my mind that he suffered from undiagnosed severe sleep apnea. One evening, three weeks before his eightieth birthday, he finished his dinner and sat down in his easy chair to watch the evening news, just as he'd done for as long as anyone could remember. After getting comfortable, he'd nod off, sitting in his chair, and start snoring.

On this particular night, he never woke up.

He had a massive heart attack, and died "peacefully" in his sleep.

Cerebrovascular disease refers to a group of conditions that affect blood flow to the brain. Obstructive sleep apnea activates the sympathetic nervous system. The sympathetic nervous system, when stimulated, activates what is often termed the "fight-or-flight response," which contributes to hypertension, increased thickening of the walls of the carotid artery (major blood vessels in the neck that supply blood to the brain, neck, and face), and an increase in fibrin (a clotting material in blood).

Metabolic issues are also associated with untreated sleep apnea. Remember the "fight-or-flight" hormone, cortisol, mentioned earlier? Elevated levels of cortisol associated with sleep apnea can negatively impact the hormone levels of leptin, the hormone that tells the brain to let us know that we're full, and ghrelin, the hormone which makes people feel hungry. When our stress levels are elevated due to high levels of cortisol, and our leptin and ghrelin hormone levels are negatively affected by lack of sleep, our brain mistakenly tells us we're hungry. We often reach for a high-carb sweet treat or comfort food that gives us a boost of energy and makes us feel better. Once the rush wears off and we crash, we go to the fridge for another quick fix. We end up unthinkingly grazing throughout the day, day in and day out, with no end in sight. It's a vicious cycle that repeats itself night after night and inevitably leads to weight gain and obesity.

This unintended weight gain puts us at increased risk for any number of health issues, least of which is the increased risk of developing insulin resistance syndrome. Insulin is a hormone made by the pancreas. It allows your cells to use glucose (sugar) for energy. Insulin resistance is a condition in which the cells of the body become resistant to the hormone insulin. The cells have trouble absorbing glucose, which causes a buildup of sugar in the blood.

Insulin resistance has been associated with a higher risk of developing heart disease and the development of type 2 diabetes. Insulin resistance often doesn't trigger any noticeable symptoms, especially early on. You could be insulin resistant for years without knowing it. A study conducted at Yale University Medical School in 2007, funded by a grant from the National Institute of Health, concluded that OSA sufferers were 2.5 times more likely to develop type 2 diabetes than non-OSA sufferers. Classic diabetes symptoms include:

- Extreme thirst or hunger
- Feeling hunger even after a meal
- Frequent or increased urination
- Tingling sensations in your hands and feet
- Feeling more tired than usual

In addition to these four main categories, untreated OSA has been shown to exacerbate other medical and social conditions as well, including: depression, a decrease in cognitive learning and coping skills, headaches, early on-set Alzheimer's, certain types of cancer, glaucoma, and reduced libido. Remember the article in the *Ladies' Home Journal* mentioned earlier that called snoring the third leading cause of divorce? A team of Swedish researchers found that individuals with OSA (as defined by symptoms of snoring and day-time sleepiness) report about three times the rate of divorce of those without OSA and/or day-time sleepiness.

Believe it or not, there was even a recent study that showed sleep apnea affected your golf score. Research studied twelve golfers with moderate to severe sleep apnea and twelve golfers without sleep apnea. The sleep-apnea sufferers were treated with CPAP for six months. Each golfer then played twenty rounds of golf. The average handicap for the non-suffering control group started at 8.4 and increased to 9.2 by the end of the study. The sleep-apnea sufferers who'd been treated with CPAP saw their handicaps move from an average of 9.2 to 6.3. by the time the test was concluded—a 31% improvement. Golf seems to require precisely the skills that treatment for sleep apnea improves.

"We know that in the cognitive parameters—Vigilance, Attention Span, Memory—people with sleep apnea do poorly on these tests and improve with treatment," said the lead author of the study, Dr. Marc L. Benton, Medical Director of the Sleepwell Center of New Jersey.

The last category, mentioned at the beginning of the chapter, *societal costs*, will be addressed in the next chapter. My insurance company, as it turned out, knew a lot more about obstructive sleep apnea and the risks associated with not getting treatment than I did.

CHAPTER 14
Health Costs Aren't the Only Costs!

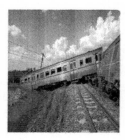

It only makes sense that when your sleep is constantly being interrupted it will take a toll on your entire body and overall health—but a tired "you" is going to have other problems as well. These problems will likely contribute to the overall increase in what are known as *societal costs* of untreated sleep apnea.

Societal costs are additional private and external costs a society must bear due to an event.

As an example, let's say you smoke. The private cost is $6.00 for a pack of cigarettes. But there are external costs to society as well. These costs include:

- Air pollution and the risks of passive smoke on others
- Litter from discarded cigarette butts
- Fires caused by improperly disposed-of cigarettes
- Health costs associated with smoking

Remember earlier in the book when we discussed excessive day-time sleepiness? You may have even taken the Epworth Sleepiness Scale Quiz to find out if you were part of the sleepy crowd. The societal costs of EDS, which is often a symptom of untreated OSA, are staggering.

A new report prepared by Frost & Sullivan and commissioned by the American Academy of Sleep Medicine has shown that the societal cost of sleep apnea in the United States is $150 billion dollars annually. The costs are broken down as follows:

- Sleep-related fatigue costs businesses in America more than $86.9 billion a year in absenteeism, workplace accidents, and lost productivity. Furthermore, looking at work-related injuries across all industries, individuals who reported disturbed sleep were nearly twice as likely to die in a work-related accident.

- Patients with OSA see the doctor twice as often and spend twice as much on medical care as those without OSA, for up to ten years prior to diagnosis. This amounts to $30 billion dollars in additional medical costs in the United States every year.
- Diagnosis and treatment would result in $100 billion in savings, the report concludes.

Additional studies provide us with additional societal costs associated with untreated sleep apnea:

- In the year 2000, more than 800,000 drivers were involved in sleep-apnea related motor vehicle accidents in the United States. These accidents resulted in the loss of life of 1,400 individuals and a monetary cost of $26.2 billion dollars a year.
- The National Transportation Safety Board (NTSB) estimates that 28% of all commercial truck drivers suffer from OSA. There are approximately 110,000 injuries and 5,000 fatalities every year involving commercial trucks. The NTSB estimated that fatigue was the probable cause of 57% of crashes that resulted in driver death. For each truck driver fatality, another 3 to 4 people were killed.
- Some additional accidents you may have heard about that have been attributed to sleep apnea include the Chernobyl nuclear reactor meltdown in 1986, and the Exxon Valdez oil spill off the coast of Southeast Alaska in 1989, where 11 million gallons of crude oil were spilled into the pristine Alaskan waters. The costs to society associated with these events were $235 billion and $7 billion, respectively. We may never know the true, long-term cost to the environment.

- On a lighter note (or maybe not if you were there), the Federal Aviation Administration (FAA) suspended two pilots who fell asleep in the cockpit and overshot their destination by fifteen miles. In 2008, the pilots of Go! Airlines 1102 failed to respond to nearly a dozen calls from air traffic controllers and repeated attempts by the flight attendants to get their attention. The captain was later diagnosed with sleep apnea. Go! Airlines was an inter-island carrier operating out of Hilo, Hawaii at the time.

Theses external societal costs have become so great that the Federal Motor Carrier Safety Administration (FMCSA) and the Federal Railroad Administration (FRA), who oversee the commercial trucking and railroad industries respectively, are considering establishing guidelines for the mandatory testing for OSA in commercial truck drivers and railroad engineers. The following incidents are just two of the many examples given for this potential policy change:

- On July 26, 2000, the driver of a tractor-trailer traveling on Interstate 40 near Jackson, Tennessee, collided with a Tennessee Highway Patrol vehicle trailing construction vehicles, killing the state trooper inside. The tractor-trailer then traveled across the median and collided with a Chevrolet Blazer heading in the opposite direction, seriously injuring the driver of the Blazer. The tractor-trailer driver was 5'11", weighed 358 pounds, and had been diagnosed with and undergone surgery for OSA, but had not indicated either the diagnosis or the surgery on examinations for medical certification. The NTSB found that the driver's unreported OSA, untreated hypothyroidism, or complications from either or both conditions predisposed him to impairment or incapacitation, including falling asleep at the wheel while driving. The NTSB determined the probable cause of the accident was the driver's incapacitation, which resulted from the failure of the medical certification process to detect and remove a medically unfit driver from service.

- On December 1, 2013, at approximately 7:20 a.m. EST, southbound Metro-North Railroad passenger train 8808 derailed as it approached the Spuyten Duyvil Station in New York City. All passenger cars and the locomotive derailed, and, as a result, four passengers died and at least 61 passengers were injured. The train was traveling at 82 mph when it derailed in a section of curved track where the maximum authorized speed was 30 mph. Following the accident, the engineer reported that: (1) he felt dazed just before the derailment; and (2) his wife had previously complained about his snoring. The engineer then underwent a sleep evaluation, which identified excessive day-time sleepiness, followed by a sleep - study, which diagnosed severe OSA. Based on its investigation of the derailment, the NTSB concluded that the engineer had multiple OSA risk factors, such as obesity, male gender, snoring, complaints of fatigue, and excessive day-time sleepiness. Even though the engineer exhibited these OSA risk factors, neither his personal healthcare provider nor his Metro-North occupational health evaluations had screened the engineer for OSA. The NTSB determined that the probable cause of the accident was the "engineer's noncompliance with the 30-mph speed restriction because he had fallen asleep due to undiagnosed severe obstructive sleep apnea, exacerbated by a recent circadian rhythm shift required by his work schedule."

- The FAA, which is responsible for all commercial and private aviation, is considering implementing similar guidelines for all commercial and private pilots.

CHAPTER 15
If Not CPAP, Then What?

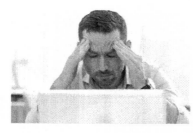 One evening, about a year after my talk with my insurance agent, I looked down at my young daughter asleep in her crib. If I wanted to watch her grow up into a beautiful young woman, if I wanted the chance to walk her down the aisle on her wedding day, I needed to take care of my sleep apnea. The next morning, I made another appointment with the sleep doctor.

While sitting in his office waiting for him to arrive, I noticed a small mouth-guard-looking thing sitting on his desk, but didn't give it a second thought. When he came in and sat down, I told him the whole story, starting with giving up on the CPAP and finishing with my insurance company conversation. I sheepishly admitted that I now understood how serious obstructive sleep apnea was, and that I was willing to give treatment another shot—as long as it wasn't CPAP.

He looked at me and said, "There are no other options for you. Your condition is too serious."

What I didn't know was that, like most sleep doctors, before my sleep doctor was a sleep doctor, he was a pulmonologist. A pulmonologist is a medical specialist who deals with the causes, diagnosis, and treatment of diseases affecting the lungs. His training had focused on, and was limited to, continuous positive airway pressure—CPAP. You know the old saying, "If the only tool you have is a hammer, everything looks like a nail"? You get the picture.

Looking down at his desk, I again saw the mouth-guard thing.

"What's that?" I asked.

"It's an oral appliance," he responded. "It sometimes works for people with very mild sleep apnea, but it would never work for you. You're too sick."

I asked, "Can I try it?"

He just repeated himself: "I told you it won't work for you!"

"Is there anything I can do to convince you to let me try it?" I asked, almost pleadingly.

He thought for a moment and said, "Go home, lose thirty pounds, and I'll let you try it."

As a side note, my sleep doctor's governing body, the American Academy of Sleep Medicine, has come a long way since my doctor's appointment in 2008. Their guidelines for the treatment of OSA, published in 2015, are summarized here:

- Oral appliance therapy should be prescribed for adult patients with OSA, rather than no treatment at all.
- Oral appliance therapy should also be offered to those patients who prefer an alternative therapy to CPAP, and for those patients who are intolerant of CPAP.
- Consult a qualified dentist who uses a custom device which can be calibrated, rather than non-custom appliances.
- Trained dentists should provide oversight to manage any dental-related side effects.
- Follow-up testing by sleep physicians is recommended once oral device calibration is completed.
- A periodic follow up with both physicians and dentists is recommended, as opposed to no follow up.

CHAPTER 16
Alternative Treatment Options

Unfortunately, the physician's office you end up in might determine which treatment options you are given. This shouldn't be the case in 2016, but people have biases based on their education and experience—even medical professionals. What I'm going to share with you are all the treatment options that I'm aware of, without bias.

- **Weight Loss**—As we've previously discussed, and the comment from my sleep doctor about losing thirty pounds suggests, excessive weight and/or obesity is a major contributor to the onset of sleep apnea. Weight loss can decrease the severity of sleep apnea, and in some cases eliminate it altogether.

- **Positional Therapy**—For a small percentage of individuals (less than 5%) who have sleep apnea, positional therapy works. If you only stop breathing while you're on your back, a product like the SlumberBump when strapped around your torso keeps you from sleeping on you back.

- **CPAP, Bi-PAP & Auto PAP**—These all work on the same principle of maintaining on open airway through the use of blown air.

- **The Winx Sleep Therapy System**—This is a CPAP running in reverse. The airway is maintained by a machine which slowly sucks air out of your mouth. This technology is fairly new.

- **Surgery**—There are multiple surgical procedures that can be successful in treating sleep apnea. They can be as aggressive as orthognathic surgery, where your lower jaw is broken and moved forward to prevent your airway from collapsing, or as benign as the Pillar Procedure. During a Pillar Procedure the surgeon implants biocompatible rods under the skin on the roof of your mouth. This procedure stretches the soft tissue, which prevents it from blocking the airway while you sleep. A uvulopalatopharyngoplasty, or UPPP, is the most common surgery used in treating sleep apnea. Typically, an ear, nose, and throat (ENT) doctor preforms this procedure. It consists of removing all the soft tissue from your mouth and throat, including your tonsils, adenoids, uvula, and pharyngeal tissue. Lastly, and fairly new, is hypoglossal nerve stimulation surgery. During this procedure an electrode is attached to the hypoglossal nerve, located at the base of the tongue. The electrode is attached via a wire to a small battery implanted in your chest. Whenever your tongue begins to slide back while you sleep, the electrode gives the hypoglossal nerve a shock which moves the tongue forward.

- **Oral Appliance Therapy**—OAT consists of a custom-made "mouth-guard" fitted by a dentist. The appliance fits over your upper and lower teeth, and is positioned so that it moves and holds your lower jaw slightly forward while you sleep, keeping your airway open.

WARNING: IF THIS IS THE TREATMENT ALTERNATIVE YOU CHOSE, BEWARE. ALL APPLIANCES ARE NOT CREATED EQUALLY. DO NOT BUY AN ORAL APPLIANCE ON LATENIGHT TELEVISION, NO MATTER HOW GOOD THEY LOOK OR WHAT KIND OF A DEAL IS OFFERED. THESE DEVICES WILL LIKELY CAUSE MORE HARM THAN GOOD. GET YOUR CUSTOM-MADE DEVICE FROM A DENTIST. PREFERABLY ONE WHO'S HAD SPECIALIZED TRAINING IN TREATING OBSTRUCTIVE SLEEP APNEA.

(See the resources section at the end of the book for recommendations.)

CHAPTER 17
Back to My Story

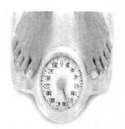

I took him up on his offer and lost the weight.

Six weeks later I was back at the sleep doctor's office, having held up my end of the bargain. I'd lost thirty-six pounds and was ready to try oral appliance therapy (OAT), which was the official terminology for the "mouth-guard" still sitting on his desk. He congratulated me on my weight loss and then proceeded to tell me that OAT still wouldn't work for me—due to my severe sleep apnea. I reminded him of our deal and he reluctantly wrote me a prescription for an oral device, with one condition: I had to have a follow-up efficacy sleep study three months after my appliance was delivered. I agreed and out the door I went.

One of the many benefits I discovered during my career was that many of my dental customers had become my friends, and one had even become my wife. Carrie is one of the most talented dentists I've ever met, and by far the prettiest.

During my struggles with OSA, she had taken a continuing education course from one of the true leaders in dental sleep medicine, Dr. Jonathan Parker. She came home from the course with a new passion—the treatment of sleep apnea with an oral appliance, which she implemented into her practice.

As she began treating patients in her own practice, the satisfaction she felt in treating these patients intensified her passion for it tenfold. She would come home at night with stories about patients who'd come into the office after being treated and tell her how much she'd both changed and improved their lives.

This continued until the summer of 2015, when she sold her general practice, and together with another dental sleep medicine believer, opened a practice limited to the treatment of OSA.

More and more dentists around the United States are experiencing the same satisfaction as my wife and are doing the same thing. Any dentist can provide this service, but remember—you are dealing with a potentially life-threatening medical condition. If oral appliance therapy is something you're considering, I would strongly encourage you to search out one of these passionate individuals. You can find one of these dentists in your area at www.aadsm.org. Under the "Patient Resources" heading you'll find additional information about Snoring, OSA, and other interesting topics. You'll also see a "Find a Dentist" tab—click on it, enter your zip code, hit search, and a list of dentists in your area will pop up. The dentists on the list whose names are Gold Starred have earned diplomate status in the AADSM. These doctors have sat and passed a rigorous written exam, as well as treated, documented, and submitted the outcomes of numerous patients to the American Academy of Dental Sleep Medicine Board. Simply put: these diplomates are the best of the best.

There are over one hundred oral appliances currently FDA-approved for OSA, but they all do the same thing. They move the lower jaw forward, and prevent it from sliding back during the night while you sleep. Some do it better than others, and some are more comfortable than others. You and a knowledgeable dental sleep medicine specialist should look at several available options and determine together which device would be appropriate for you. Several things to remember when choosing a device are:

- It must be FDA-approved for the treatment of OSA, not just snoring.
- It must be custom-made for your mouth.
- The mechanism that moves your lower jaw forward must be adjustable.
- Most of the better devices come with a three-year warranty.

I've tried many devices over the last five years, and have had the greatest success with the dorsal design, because it's comfortable in my mouth. Comfort is key. If it's not comfortable you won't use it.

CHAPTER 18
Me and My Oral Appliance

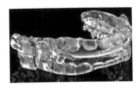 With my prescription in hand I went directly to my wife's office. My experience there is an example of what you might experience yourself, so listen closely!

The dentist will first do a comprehensive exam to make sure that you're a good candidate for oral appliance therapy. Remember this: even though you have a prescription for an oral appliance from a sleep physician, sleep physicians aren't dentists. Dentists are doctors who specialize in the mouth. Prior to making your custom appliance, they may take X-rays to look at your airway. They will check for cavities and/or crowns that should be treated, and they will check for periodontal disease, which can lead to tooth mobility. Things that turn up during your initial exam may have to be dealt with prior to having your custom appliance fabricated.

Once the exam is completed, the dentist will take impressions of your upper and lower teeth and measure your bite. This information will then be sent to an FDA-certified oral appliance manufacturer. The lab will manufacture your custom appliance and send it back to your dentist for the initial fitting. This process usually takes about three weeks.

At this point, you might be wondering about the cost of treatment.

CPAP, oral appliance therapy, and some—but not all—surgical procedures mentioned in the last chapter will usually be covered by your medical insurance or Medicare. Not all medical insurance plans are created equally, however. The dental office can, and should, help you determine if preauthorization of treatment is required, what your insurance benefits will cover, and, lastly, what your out-of-pocket cost will be, prior to treatment. In my experience, the cost of CPAP and the cost of oral appliance therapy come out to about the same amount within eighteen months of treatment. An oral appliance may cost slightly more up front, but with a CPAP, you have the recurring costs of replacing filters, hoses, and masks.

Remember, regardless of your final choice, the most expensive choice by far is to not get treated.

I returned to my dentist in three weeks to pick up my oral appliance. I tried it and it fit like a glove. At this point, different dentists may vary their protocols slightly. In my case, my device was set at my habitual or normal bite the first week to allow me to get used to having something in my mouth while I slept. Other doctors may choose a different starting point or approach, but in the end they should all reach the same desired outcome.

It took me about a week to be able to leave my appliance in my mouth all night. The first night, it was in for about four hours. Each night I could tolerate it a little bit longer. Once I was comfortable with it, with the help of my dentist I began to gradually move my lower jaw forward. The amount of movement required and the time it takes to properly adjust an appliance for a patient will vary, and should be done with the dentist's guidance. Over the course of approximately three weeks, my lower jaw was being protruded, or moved forward, an average of one millimeter a week. At the end of three weeks my lower jaw had been moved forward three millimeters, or approximately .12 inches.

While sleeping with my jaw in this position I wasn't snoring, getting up throughout the night to use the bathroom, or—most importantly—taking those afternoon naps anymore. Each morning when I got up I'd remove my appliance. After eight hours with it in my mouth, my bite would feel different. Within fifteen minutes, however, my bite returned to normal. This small inconvenience was well worth it. Finally, after thirty years, I was waking up every morning well rested and ready for a productive day.

It was time to see the sleep doctor again.

CHAPTER 19
My Final Results

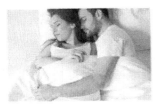 I sat in my doctor's office, with my oral appliance in my pocket. Based on how I felt, I knew my appliance was working. I was even dreaming, which I couldn't remember ever doing.

We dream when we are in a sleep cycle called REM, or rapid eye movement. Unfortunately, the REM cycle is also when OSA occurs most frequently. Because of the severity of my initial condition I seldom experienced REM sleep, and when I did it was short-lived, which explained why I didn't dream.

Even though I was sure I was sleeping soundly, only another sleep test would prove it to my doctor. Thankfully, he agreed that a home sleep study, rather than another PSG, would be sufficient to determine if my appliance was working or not. Just to be sure, he had me use the machine for two nights, which was fine with me.

I took the HST home and, following the instructions, used it over the next two nights. I returned the HST to his office on Monday morning and scheduled an appointment for the end of the week to go over the results.

He began our Friday conversation by stating, "I'm glad I had you use the HST for two nights, because I wouldn't have believed the results if it had only been one night of data."

It turns out that my AHI had gone from a 73 to below a 5 for two consecutive nights. I couldn't decide if I was mad at him or not. He'd made me jump through a lot of hoops before I finally found a treatment for my OSA that worked, and that I could tolerate. I quickly decided it wasn't worth the effort of getting mad. I had my appliance, I was sleeping like a baby, still had my pills for restless leg, and my wife was sleeping soundly as well (no more bruised ribs!).

I've continued to wear my appliance every night for the last five years. If I've had a few drinks or have added a few pounds, the snoring comes back, and my wife now politely asks me to adjust my appliance. Once the weight comes off, I adjust it back.

It has been a life-changing experience for me. I no longer suffer from excessive day-time sleepiness, my blood pressure is down, and I've maintained my weight loss. I now feel confident that I'll be around to watch my daughter grow up and become a beautiful young woman. All thanks to a little, plastic "mouth-guard" sitting on my doctor's desk.

CHAPTER 20
Pregnancy and Menopause

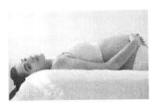 New research on obstructive sleep apnea continues to be published regularly, particularly regarding women and children. Studies now show that pregnant women are more susceptible to the onset of sleep apnea than women who aren't pregnant. Excess weight gain during pregnancy puts women at risk. Moms-to-be who have gestational diabetes are also at higher risk of having sleep apnea. Gestational diabetes develops during pregnancy. When you're pregnant, hormonal changes make your cells less responsive to insulin. For most of us this isn't a problem: when the body needs insulin, the pancreas secretes more of it—but if the pancreas can't keep up with demand during pregnancy, your blood glucose levels rise too high, resulting in gestational diabetes. Between 2–10% of expectant mothers develop this condition.

It's also believed that all pregnant women have an increased risk of OSA, due to higher levels of estrogen. When estrogen levels increase during pregnancy, the mucus membranes lining the airway can begin to swell, restricting airflow, which over time lowers your blood-oxygen levels. The less oxygen you breathe in each night, the less oxygen you and your unborn baby get.

Pregnant women with sleep apnea are more likely to suffer from preeclampsia as well. Preeclampsia is also known as pregnancy-induced hypertension (PIH), or toxemia. Toxemia is a disorder that generally develops late in pregnancy (after week 20) and is characterized by a sudden onset of high blood pressure. If left untreated, this can be dangerous for both mom and baby. Unmanaged preeclampsia can prevent the developing fetus from getting enough blood and oxygen, damage the mother's liver and kidneys, and, in rare cases, progress to eclampsia, a much more serious condition involving seizures.

At the other end of the spectrum are menopausal women. Menopause is a time of major hormonal, physical, and psychological change for women. Menopause has been linked to an increase in OSA as well. Although unconfirmed, the most likely cause of premenopausal- or menopausal-onset OSA is the decrease in estrogen and progesterone, which occurs during menopause. Higher levels of these hormones protect women prior to the onset of menopause by maintaining the airway and keeping it from collapsing.

CHAPTER 21
To the Parents of Patients

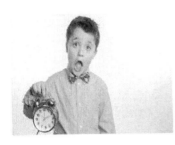

This chapter was by far the hardest to write, but it's also the most important. Everything you've read so far pales in comparison to what's in this chapter, especially if you have a young son or daughter who might also be suffering from undiagnosed, or misdiagnosed, sleep apnea. Until recently, the medical community thought that OSA was a condition that only affected adults. Pediatricians, pediatric otolaryngologists (ear, nose, and throat doctors), pediatric dentists, and orthodontists see children every day that are suffering from OSA and they don't realize it.

These healthcare providers typically only hear about the daytime symptoms. What's happening at night is, more than likely, not part of the conversation with Mom or Dad. Unfortunately, the signs of sleep apnea that are apparent during the day mimic another very common diagnosis: ADHD. When children get tired, unlike adults, they become hyperactive, impulsive, and inattentive. These are classic signs of attention deficit hyperactive disorder, or ADHD. The Center for Disease Control and Prevention (CDC) reported that "Nearly six million children in America were diagnosed with ADHD in 2011—a 43% increase from 2003." With this diagnosis comes a prescription for stimulant drugs such as Ritalin, which, for a child with sleep apnea, only makes things worse.

Sleep disorders, and specifically sleep apnea, are thought to affect approximately 1–3% of otherwise healthy children under the age of eight. The actual number of kids suffering from sleep apnea is difficult to pin down. Numerous studies have been conducted and the results vary significantly due to the way the studies were designed. What we do know is that kids shouldn't snore—ever.

According to an article published by the American Thoracic Society that conducted a meta-analysis, or review, of all studies related to the prevalence of pediatric OSA, the numbers were all over the board. In studies where parents were asked if their kids snore "always," the reported number ranged from 1.5% to 6.2%. When the question was changed to "often," the number increased to a range of 3.2% to 14.8%. Using mathematical formulas to even out the results, it was determined that 7.45% of children snore.

The study also looked at parent-reported apneic events, or times when they witnessed their child stop breathing during sleep. Again, averaging all the various studies, it was determined that approximately 4% of children experienced apneic events.

Children and teens with sleep apnea might seem to be sleeping a lot, but their sleep is constantly disturbed by micro arousals, or turbulence in their brain waves. In effect, these kids are as sleep deprived as people who only get four to five hours of sleep a night.

In addition to snoring, choking, or gasping for air during sleep, you should be aware of the following signs of a child who might be suffering from OSA:

- Mouth breathing
- Dark circles under the eyes
- Chronic congestion
- Overweight or obesity
- Bed wetting
- Nightmares
- Headaches
- Restless sleep
- Large tonsils and/or adenoids
- Chronic runny noses
- Frequent upper airway infections
- Earaches
- Bruxism

Research has shown that there is a strong correlation between young children and adolescents who get less than optimal sleep and the development of obesity. Snoring, mouth breathing, and sleep apnea can also lead to serious behavioral, emotional, and social consequences in children. These include hyperactivity, emotional issues such as anxiety and depression, peer relationship problems, and conduct problems, such as following the rules and inappropriate social interactions.

Evidence from a study conducted at the University of Arizona showed children with breathing problems as early as six months of age had a 50% increased risk of developing behavioral problems by age seven. They were also three times more likely to have school grades of C or lower. The social and emotional problems associated with sleep apnea include low self-esteem and bullying. Children often tease and bully their overweight peers, who then suffer from lowered self-esteem and depression.

At one extreme, these problems may lead to children acting out and disrupting classrooms. At the other extreme, they may socially withdraw. Untreated sleep apnea in children sets them up for a lifetime of struggle. The sooner the condition is identified and properly treated, the less impactful the negative effects will be.

The treatment options for children differ from those for adults. Although CPAP therapy can be used if the child will tolerate it, the most common treatment for children is a surgical procedure called an adenotonsillectomy—the surgical removal of the tonsils and adenoids. This procedure opens an otherwise compromised airway. Unfortunately, in some children the adenoids grow back. If it's determined that the nose or nasal passages are contributing factors, an anti-inflammatory corticosteroid may be recommended.

One more thing to consider. The American Association of Orthodontics estimates that at any given time over four million people in the US are undergoing orthodontic treatment. Why bring up orthodontics? It's reasonable to assume that many of these four million patients are children. It's also reasonable to assume that a portion of these children are seeing orthodontists who still believe that the best way to correct an over-crowded mouth is to extract or pull teeth, giving the remaining teeth more room to move and straighten out. The unintended consequence of this treatment is the narrowing of the patients' upper and lower arches. Narrowed arches leave less room for the tongue, causing it to fall back at night, reducing the airway.

The take-away from this chapter is simply this: if you have a child suffering from any of the above-mentioned symptoms, you must be their advocate. If a pediatrician or an ENT tells you not to worry about your child's abnormally large tonsils and/or uvula because they'll grow into them, find a new doctor. If an orthodontist wants to remove teeth to create space, get a second opinion. No one else but you can save your child from a lifetime of preventable challenges.

I've experienced much of this chapter firsthand. My daughter, who's now nine, was diagnosed with OSA two years ago. Although my wife and I are intimately involved in the world of sleep apnea, as a professional and a patient respectively, we missed some signs and symptoms. Luckily for us, my daughter sees a great pediatrician who mentioned that her tonsils seemed large.

Suddenly, the possibility of OSA was like a light bulb turning on. Many of the issues we were experiencing with our daughter might be directly linked to undiagnosed OSA!

This revelation led us to an ENT at a children's hospital who removed her adenoids and shaved her tonsils. Within weeks we had a happier, healthier, more attentive, and well-adjusted daughter, both at home and at school. She's continued to improve in all facets of her life, and has just started palatal expansion treatment with the orthodontist, where, with the use of a palatal expander, my daughter's upper arch is slowly widened, giving her tongue more space. I can't thank Dr. Larsen enough for the care she provided for our family.

CHAPTER 22
Conclusion

We've reached the end of my journey so far, but I won't stop. Like every medical condition, the research on obstructive sleep apnea continues to evolve, and as a patient, and a patient advocate, I'll continue to learn.

I hope that what you've read has been enlightening. It's a tragedy that so many people continue to suffer from a medical condition that's so easily treated and managed. If you recognize yourself in parts of my story don't ignore the warning signs. If you realize that a loved one may be suffering unknowingly, let them know. You could be saving a life. The following list is a recap of the important "take home" points to remember. Share it with a friend.

- The human body needs restful sleep to function efficiently.
- A large percentage of the population isn't getting an adequate amount of sleep. This may be by choice, or it may be a medical condition.
- Snoring and obstructive sleep apnea is more common than most people realize, including healthcare providers, which contributes to a high percentage of sufferers remaining undiagnosed.
- Untreated obstructive sleep apnea can lead to a laundry list of associated diseases and medical conditions.
- Your dentist might be where your OSA is first identified, but a diagnosis must come from a sleep physician.
- Sleep apnea is a medical condition that typically isn't cured, but managed over a lifetime.
- Although CPAP is still considered the gold standard for treating sleep apnea, there are other treatment

alternatives. Take a proactive approach regarding your options, because the worst option is no treatment at all.

- Getting appropriate treatment to manage your sleep apnea will have a profound impact on your health, happiness, and well-being.

- PLEASE, PLEASE, PLEASE, if your child is showing any signs or symptoms of sleep apnea, don't ignore it—let their pediatrician know your concerns. If they dismiss them or immediately jump to the diagnosis of ADHD, get a second or a third opinion.

After reading this book, you can now consider yourself an expert on snoring and obstructive sleep apnea. Chances are very good that you know more about OSA than your primary care doctor and general dentist combined. In order to get the proper treatment you need, you may have to educate them on sleep apnea. Take what you've learned in this book, along with your STOPBang and Epworth Sleepiness scores, and start a dialogue with one or both of them. If you don't get the results you want, get a second opinion (see Glossary & Resources), or, better yet, get them a copy of this book to read themselves. Not only will you be helping yourself, but you'll be helping the other undiagnosed patients in their practices as well.

Sweet dreams!

Glossary and Resources

A

Adenoids—a patch of tissue that sit in the back of the nasal cavity. Abnormally large adenoids often obstruct breathing through the nose.

Adenotonsillectomy—a surgical procedure where the adenoids are removed and the tonsils are either shaved or removed.

Adrenaline—a hormone secreted by the adrenal gland during times of stress, causing a heightened state of arousal.

Advocate—a person who writes, speaks, pleads, and argues for a person who is incapable of defending themselves.

Apnea Hypopnea Index, or AHI—an index used to determine the severity of an individual's obstructive sleep apnea. It is the combined number of apnea and hypopnea events per hour of sleep.

American Academy of Sleep Medicine, or AASM—a sleep medicine association for professionals dedicated to the treatment of sleep disorders such as sleep apnea and insomnia. www.aasm.org

American Academy of Dental Sleep Medicine, or AADSM—a sister organization of the AASM, made up of dental professionals dedicated to the use of oral appliance therapy in the treatment of obstructive sleep apnea. www.aadsm.org

American Thoracic Society, or ATS—a nonprofit organization focused on improving care for pulmonary diseases, critical illnesses, and sleep-related breathing disorders.

Anesthesiologist—a physician trained in administering drugs or other agents to patients during surgery to prevent pain.

Apnea—a pause in breathing that lasts a minimum of ten seconds and is associated with a 3% drop in oxygen in the blood. When combined with hypopneas events during a one-hour period of sleep, the combined numbers produce an AHI score.

Attention Deficit Hyperactive Disorder, or ADHD—commonly diagnosed in children as a brain disorder marked by an ongoing pattern of inattention and/or hyperactivity and impulsive behavior.

B

Barbiturates—medications used for sedation, which have largely been phased out as sleep aids due to serious side effects, including addiction and withdrawal.

Benzodiazepines—medications prescribed to treat or relieve anxiety. Some work as muscle relaxants.

Biological Needs—basic needs like food, water, and air that humans need to survive.

Body Mass Index, or BMI—an index of height-to-weight ratio to determine if a person is overweight or obese. A BMI calculator can be found at www.smartbmicalculator.com.

Bruxism—also known as "tooth grinding," it is the medical term for grinding or clenching your teeth. 25 million Americans unconsciously grind their teeth and/or clench their jaw, either while awake or asleep. Bruxism is often caused by stress or anxiety.

C

Cardiovascular Disease—generally refers to conditions or diseases affecting the blood vessels and/or heart, including high blood pressure and heart attack.

Carotid Arteries—located on each side of your neck, they are the major blood vessels that supply blood to your brain.

Center for Disease Control and Prevention, or CDC—a federal agency that conducts and supports health promotion, prevention, and preparedness activities in the United States with the goal of improving overall public health.

Cerebrovascular Disease—refers to a group of conditions that affect blood flow to the brain. This can include thickening of the walls of the carotid arteries and an increase in fibrinogen.

Circadian Rhythm or Circadian Clock—often referred to as the "body clock," it tells our bodies when to sleep, get up, and eat. This internal clock can be effected by environmental cues, like sunlight and temperature. (see *Melatonin*)

Cognitive Learning—a basic function of learning based on how a person processes and understands information. It includes problem-solving skills, memory retention, and thinking skills.

Composite Fillings—a resin-based material used to fill cavities.

Comorbidity—the presence of one or more additional diseases or disorders occurring simultaneously with a primary disease.

Corticosteroid—a man-made drug that when inhaled suppresses inflammation in the airway. They mimic the effects of hormones your body produces naturally.

Cortisol—a hormone commonly associated with "fight or flight," which can become elevated in response to physical or psychological stress. Elevated levels of Cortisol suppress the immune system, which keeps us healthy and effects metabolism, causing weight gain.

Continuous Positive Air Pressure, or CPAP—a machine which is attached to a patient via a hose and mask. The machine blows air down the airway, preventing it from collapsing during sleep.

D

Durable Medical Equipment, or DME—a company who supplies medical equipment such as wheel chairs, oxygen, crutches, and CPAPs to patients.

Dorsal Design Oral Appliance—a design where either the upper or lower appliance has a component that looks like a dorsal (or "shark's") fin.

E

Eclampsia—the result of uncontrolled or unresolved preeclampsia, a condition characterized by high blood pressure, swelling, and protein in the urine.

Empress Porcelain—a special porcelain used to make crowns without metal reinforcement. The lack of metal makes the crown appear more natural.

Epidemic—a widespread occurrence that affects a community at any given time.

Epworth Sleepiness Scale—a questionnaire that determines if an individual is suffering from excessive day-time sleepiness.

Estrogen—a hormone which increases during pregnancy. When estrogen levels get too high, the tissue lining the airway begins to swell, restricting airflow, which over time can reduce the oxygen levels in the blood, negatively affecting the mother and fetus.

Excessive Day-time Sleepiness—a persistent sleepiness, and often a general lack of energy, during the day after getting apparently adequate or even prolonged nighttime sleep.

F

Federal Aviation Administration, or FAA—a government agency primarily responsible for the advancement, safety, and regulation of civil aviation, as well as overseeing the air traffic control system in the United States.

Federal Motor Carrier Safety Administration, or FMCSA—a federal agency within the US Department of Transportation which enforces safety regulations, hazardous materials regulations, drug and alcohol regulations, medical regulations, and hours of service behind the wheel, for the commercial trucking industry.

Federal Railroad Administration, or FRA—acting within the US Department of Transportation, the FRA holds the same authority over the railroads in the United States as the FMCSA has for commercial trucking.

Fibrin (also called Factor Ia)—a protein in the blood plasma that is essential for blood coagulation or clotting.

G

Gestational Diabetes—develops during pregnancy, when hormonal changes make cells less responsive to insulin. If the pancreas can't keep up with the increased demand for insulin, blood sugar levels rise too high, resulting in gestational diabetes.

H

Home Sleep Test or Out of Center Sleep Test (HST or OCST)—a sleep test which is self-administered by the patient in his or her on bed.

Hypoglossal Nerve Stimulation Surgery—a procedure where an electrode is implanted at the hypoglossal nerve at the base of the tongue. A wire is then run from the nerve to a battery implanted in the patient's chest. As the patient falls asleep and the tongue begins to fall back a small shock hits the back of the tongue, causing it to remain forward.

Hypopnea—a 50% reduction in airflow lasting longer than 10 seconds. When combined with apnea events during a one-hour period of sleep, the combined numbers produce an AHI score.

I

Incisal Edge Sleep—a Facebook page dedicated to sleep issues, including obstructive sleep apnea.

M

Melatonin—a hormone which helps regulate the time we go to sleep and wake up and can be affected by the presence of light.

Meta-Analysis—uses a statistical approach to combine the results of multiple independent studies in an effort to improve estimates of the size of the effect and/or to resolve uncertainty when studies or reports disagree.

Metabolism—the sum of the physical and chemical processes in which an organism uses food, water, etc., to grow, heal, and make energy to survive.

Menopause—a time in a woman's life of major hormonal, physical, and psychological change. Menopause has been linked to an increased risk of obstructive sleep apnea. Although unconfirmed, the most likely cause is the decrease in estrogen and progesterone, associated with menopause.

Micro Arousals—an abrupt change from sleep to wakefulness, or from a "deeper" sleep stage of non-REM sleep to a "lighter" stage. A partial awakening from sleep.

N

National Sleep Foundation, or NSF—dedicated to the health and well-being of people through sleep research. More information can be found at www.sleepfoundation.org.

National Transportation Safety Board, or NTSB—an independent federal agency charged with investigating every civil aviation accident in the United States and significant accidents in other modes of transportation, including railroad, highway, marine, and pipeline accidents.

Neurologist—a medical doctor who specializes in treating diseases of the nervous system.

New England Journal of Medicine—a well-respected medical journal in which peer-reviewed research is published.

Noncompliance—in medicine, the term, "noncompliance" is commonly used in regard to a patient who does not take a prescribed medication or follow a prescribed course of treatment.

O

Obesity—an abnormal accumulation of body fat, usually 20% or more, over an individual's ideal body weight.

Obstructive Sleep Apnea, or OSA—a potentially serious sleep disorder. It causes breathing to repeatedly stop and start during sleep.

Occupational Safety and Health Administration, or OSHA—a government agency that sets and monitors guidelines for worker safety across all industries.

Opiates—medications used to treat pain. They can cause sleepiness, irregular breathing, and shallow breaths.

Oral Appliance—a custom-made dental device, typically made of acrylic, metal, plastic, or nylon, used during sleep to treat obstructive sleep apnea.

Oral Appliance Therapy—an alternative to CPAP therapy for treating obstructive sleep apnea, whereby the lower jaw of a patient is positioned slightly forward with the use of a custom-made dental appliance.

Orthodontist—a dental specialist trained to prevent, diagnose, and treat facial and dental irregularities, such as malocclusions (bad bites), through the use of treatments like braces.

Orthognathic Surgery—a surgical procedure where an oral surgeon fractures your lower jaw and repositions it forward from where it was. When the fracture heals, your lower jaw is permanently moved forward, preventing your airway from collapsing during sleep.

P

Palatal Expansion—with the use of a palatal expander placed by an orthodontist, the upper jaw is widened so that the upper and lower teeth will fit together better. This procedure is also used to give the tongue more room to move forward away from the airway.

Pediatrician—a medical doctor specializing in the treatment of children and their diseases.

Pediatric Dentist—a specialist who only treats children from infancy through the early teens.

Peer-reviewed research—research which has been checked and verified by a group of experts in the same field, prior to being published.

Pharynx—the body cavity that connects the nasal and oral cavities with the larynx and esophagus. It is commonly referred to as the throat.

Pillar Procedure—a procedure where a surgeon implants biocompatible rods under the skin of your soft palate, which is the back portion of the roof of your mouth. The rods stretch the soft tissue, preventing it from vibrating during snoring and collapsing during sleep.

Polysomnography, or PSG—a sleep study administered in a hospital or sleep lab, where the patient is monitored throughout the night by a registered sleep technician.

Positional Therapy—some people only experience sleep apnea while asleep on their back. Positional therapy uses an external device, which keeps you from sleeping in a supine position (on your back).

Preeclampsia—also known as pregnancy-induced hypertension, or toxemia, it is the sudden onset of high blood pressure. Unmanaged preeclampsia can prevent the fetus from getting enough blood and oxygen, and may lead to eclampsia.

Prevalence—a measurement of all individuals affected by a disease or condition at the same time.

Psychiatrist—a medical doctor specializing in the diagnosis and treatment of mental illness.

Pulmonologist—a medical doctor who specializes in the diagnosis and treatment of lung conditions and breathing disorders.

R

REM Sleep (Rapid Eye Movement)—a recurring period of sleep during the night, totaling about two hours, where dreaming takes place. REM is characterized by rapid periodic twitching movements of the eye muscles and other physiological changes, such as accelerated respiration and heart rate, increased brain activity, and muscle relaxation and/or paralysis. Muscle paralysis happens during this stage as a safety measure so that we don't act out what's happening in our dreams. This is the stage of sleep where episodes of sleep apnea tend to increase.

Restless Leg Syndrome, or RLS—a disorder characterized by an unpleasant tickling or twitching sensation in the leg muscles when sitting or lying down, which is relieved only by moving the legs.

Rhinitis—a common side effect of CPAP usage, nasal inflammation that results in a runny nose, congestion, nasal itching, and sneezing.

Ritalin—a central nervous system stimulant. It affects chemicals in the brain that contribute to hyperactivity and impulse control. It is often given to individuals diagnosed with ADHD.

S

Seizures—usually close to or during delivery, seizures are the most common symptom of eclampsia. Depending on what stage of pregnancy a woman is in when she becomes eclampsic, the baby may be at risk of being born prematurely, as immediate delivery is often the only treatment. Luckily, eclampsia is fairly rare, occurring in one out of every 2,000 to 3,000 pregnancies.

Sleep Deprived or Sleep Deprivation—a condition where an individual is not getting enough sleep.

Sleep Disorders—changes in sleeping patterns or habits.

Sleep Fragmentation—arousals and awakenings during the night that disrupt normal sleep.

Sleep Hygiene—a series of habits and rituals that can improve your ability to fall asleep and stay asleep for an appropriate amount of time.

Sleep Physician—a medical doctor trained in the diagnosis and treatment of sleep disturbances and disorders.

Sleep Onset—the time it takes a person to fall asleep once they've gotten into bed.

Societal Costs—additional private and external costs associated with an event or a behavior that society must pay for.

Soft Palate—the soft tissue which makes up the back portion of the roof of the mouth. It differs from the hard palate, which is the front portion of the roof of the mouth, in that it does not contain bone.

STOPBang Questionnaire—an eight-question survey that predicts an individual's risk of having obstructive sleep apnea.

Sleep Stages—humans pass through stages of sleep during the night. These stages progress in a cycle from Stage 1 through REM, and then begin again back at Stage 1. A complete sleep cycle lasts 90–120 minutes depending on the individual. Stage 1 is very light, easily disrupted sleep. Stage 2 is the stage where we spend most of the night. It is characterized by deeper sleep, a slower heart rate, and a decrease in body temperature. Stage 3 is the deepest stage of non-REM sleep. The sleeper is largely unaware of and unresponsive to the outside environment. (see *REM Sleep* for definition of this stage)

T

Tissue Fluorescence—a process where a specific wavelength of light is shone in the mouth. The light causes the skin to glow an "apple green" color if it's healthy. Unhealthy skin appears dark.

Titration or Calibration Sleep Study—a type of in-lab sleep study used to calibrate CPAP therapy. The sleep technician adjusts the air pressure of the CPAP until a patient's sleep apnea is controlled.

Tonsils—a pair of soft tissue masses located at the rear of the throat. Large tonsils can compromise the airway in children.

Turbulence—a violent, unsteady, or increased movement of air or water.

U

Undiagnosed—an individual who is unaware that they are suffering from a medical condition or disease. A disease that has not been diagnosed or recognized.

Upper and Lower Arches—your crescent-shaped upper and lower jaws, which hold your teeth in place.

Uvulopalatopharyngoplasty Surgery, or UPPP—a surgical procedure done by an otolaryngologist (ear, nose, and throat doctor) who removes or remodels the tonsils, adenoids, uvula, soft palate, and pharynx using a laser or scalpel.

Uvula—a fleshy extension at the back of the soft palate that hangs down the throat

V

VELscope—stands for "Visually Enhanced Lesion" scope. The technology developed by LED Medical Diagnostics to show dentists unhealthy tissue in the mouth that they couldn't see with the naked eye. (see *Tissue Fluorescence*)

W

Winx Sleep Therapy System—works like a CPAP in reverse, gently sucking the soft tissue forward in the mouth while the patient sleeps.

Proof

Made in the USA
Charleston, SC
09 December 2016